YOUR GUIDE TO MAKING FRIENDS

Simple tips to expand your social circle

Written by Joachim Gaulin

Translated by Rebecca Neal

Health and Wellbeing 50MINUTES.com

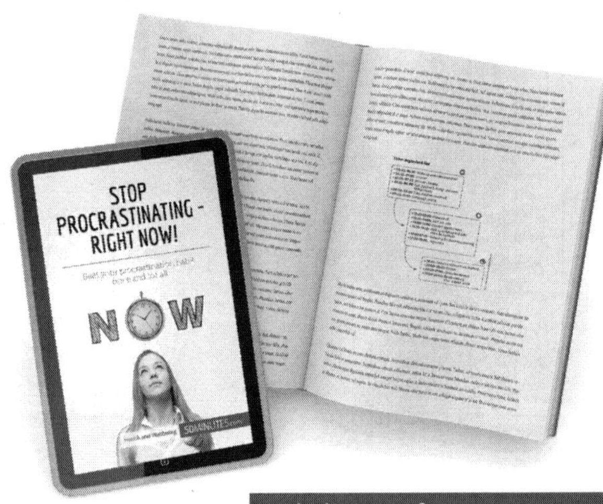

50MINUTES.com

HEALTH AND WELLBEING
WITHOUT THE HEADACHE

STOP
PROCRASTINATING –
RIGHT NOW!

NOW

Make learning fun!

Learn to love yourself

Dealing with bullying at school

Your guide to making friends

www.50minutes.com

Is it possible to make and keep friends if I move a lot?

How can I keep my new friends?

YOUR GUIDE TO MAKING FRIENDS

- **Problem:** you want to expand your circle of friends but struggle to meet new people who share your interests, or you are shy and need advice to get better at talking to people who you do not know that well.
- **Aim:** to stop being lonely and meet new people to establish lasting friendships.
- **FAQs:**
  - Is it easy to make friends?
  - Is shyness an obstacle to friendship?
  - What are the main obstacles stopping us from making friends?
  - What are some tips to make new friends?
  - Where can I meet new friends?
  - Is it possible to make and keep friends if I move a lot?
  - How can I keep my new friends?

In our hyperconnected world, where everyone has contacts and acquaintances but few people they can truly count on, it is not always easy to form lasting friendships. Although many people see friendship as one of the most important things in their life, a 2015 survey by the French polling organisation TNS Sofres revealed that 7% of French people say that they have no friends.

It is true that getting out and meeting people is not always a simple task. However, sometimes all you need is a little push and a few tips to open up to others. Of course, you will need to make some effort to get into the habit of striking up a conversation with someone you do not know and to be cheerful and friendly towards the people around you, but this will only make the rewards greater. For the shyest among you, there are websites where you can meet friends. However, these sites are only a preliminary stage that will show you that you are capable of getting out and meeting people. Once you have this newfound self-confidence, you will be able to come out of your shell, open yourself up to the world and make the most of everything it has to offer.

WHY DO I STRUGGLE TO MAKE FRIENDS?

If you struggle to make friends, it is important to understand why. You may just not know where or how to meet new people, but you could also have a more general problem with relationships.

Whatever is holding you back, it is worth taking your courage in both hands, because loneliness and isolation are rarely easy to live with.

YOU LACK SELF-CONFIDENCE

A lack of confidence is probably the most common reason people struggle to establish new relationships. People with low self-esteem see themselves as inferior to other people and sometimes think that they will never amount to anything and are not good enough. This causes them to withdraw into themselves. This feeling of being out of place and of not being good enough stops them from approaching other people, particularly because they fear that they will be seen as boring and rejected.

To rediscover your lost self-esteem, you will need to be patient and focus on two essential points: letting go and tolerance, especially towards yourself. Meditation can help you with this, because it will allow you to change the way you see yourself and life in general. The people around you will also help you in your quest, because becoming aware of how much your loved ones appreciate you will allow you to regain your self-confidence.

YOU ARE SCARED OF BEING JUDGED

The fear of being judged by others and of them not liking you is linked to a lack of self-confidence and can prevent you from opening up to others. The feeling that they are looking at you can stop you from being yourself and asserting your opinion, because you are afraid of being rejected or seeming ridiculous.

Although this is an entirely normal defence mechanism, it stops you from revealing your real personality and being true to yourself. It is therefore important to be aware that, in this situation, you are your own worst enemy, and not the other person, who just wants to find out more about you. Overcoming this defence mechanism will allow you to get to know more people. To achieve this, the first things to do are to get to know yourself, discover your desires and passions, and let yourself express them. As a starting point, feel free to express your ideas about little things in a debate. Expressing yourself will enable you to develop your assertiveness and self-confidence.

YOU ARE SHY

Shyness is a problem in relationships if it is excessive or too noticeable. Some people struggle to express themselves when they are in a group because they do not like drawing attention to themselves. They are therefore often withdrawn and do not participate much in discussions.

To overcome your shyness, you could start by taking an interest in one person within your group and focusing on the things you can find out by talking to them. You could then move on to talking to other members of the group.

However, shyness is not necessarily an obstacle, and, when it is mild, it even has significant advantages. Indeed, shy people often make excellent leaders, because they know how to bring out the best in others and are more attentive to their needs. They also have impressive observation skills, which often go hand in hand with the ability to listen, an essential element of friendship.

Ultimately, it is important to remember that, unless your shyness is very acute, it is not a flaw to overcome, but a way of being that you need to harness to prevent it from being an obstacle in your social life.

YOU ARE AFRAID OF CONFLICT

You hate tension and do everything in your power to avoid causing it. As a result, you struggle to say no and tend to go along with the general opinion, even if you originally had a different viewpoint. To avoid offending other people, you prefer to sit on the fence, which can irritate some of your friends and family.

To remedy this, you need to learn to assert yourself and not be afraid of expressing your opinions, even if they are not the same as other people's. Although you may find it hard to believe, clearly (but not aggressively) stating your positions will not drive people away; on the contrary, it will allow them to get to know you and your ideals. Your friends and family can help you in this process by urging you to make decisions, even if they are not very important, and encouraging you to express your point of view.

YOU ARE AUTHORITARIAN

It is important for you to control things and to be fair, unbiased and efficient. You are more interested and place greater trust in people who are assertive, honest and have a strong personality. You do not do anything by halves and approach everything with energy. You are generally quick to agree to help others, but you feel the need to take control of the situation and expect to be thanked for this. Although this kind of personality suits some people, others may find it infuriating, as they see it as overbearing. You are therefore alienating many people who could have become good friends.

Consequently, it is important to learn to let go and pay greater attention to others and their needs. They may feel that your way of doing things is too blunt and aggressive. Show that you are prepared to listen. This will allow you to improve your interactions with other people naturally.

YOU ARE A PESSIMIST

People with underdeveloped social lives are often pessimists. This is frequently linked to a lack of self-confidence, which fuels the problem. People then tend to only see the negative side of things and to imagine, for one reason or another, that their relationships are doomed to failure before they have even got off the ground. All this impacts the image that we convey of ourselves: other people see us as bitter, anxious and even aggressive, which makes it harder to make new friends.

It is therefore important to work on the way you look at life. Most of the time, it is possible to take something positive from every situation. Try to find this positive side and learn to enjoy life's little pleasures. It will take time for you to really appreciate them, but this will only make you happier in the end. By presenting a positive image of yourself, you will encourage others to come to you.

YOU HAVE TRUST ISSUES

You may have had your fingers burnt by previous bad experiences, which stops you from trusting others. Maybe a friend disappointed you by not being there when you needed them or at an important time in your life. Even worse, they may have betrayed you. Alternatively, perhaps a person who seemed nice really only cared about what you could do for them. Do not dwell on this bad impression. Although some of your relationships did not turn out well, you can tell yourself that these bad experiences are not inevitable. In any case, try to move forward and do not turn your back on other people.

YOU DO NOT HAVE TIME

When your personal life is already hectic, you often do not have time to go out and meet new people.

Indeed, you need to invest in forging new relationships. Unfortunately, we often do not have much time to devote to this, whether because of family or because of work. Nonetheless, you should try to clear a slot in your schedule at least once per week for an activity where you will be able to spend time with friends or new people. Try to do this regularly and miss it as little as possible.

METHODS AND TIPS FOR MAKING FRIENDS

WHAT IS FRIENDSHIP?

Before giving advice to open up to others and build lasting relationships, it may be useful to take a closer look at what friendship is and why it is important.

Friendship occupies an essential place in most people's lives, and they generally consider it beneficial to their happiness and personal balance. According to one survey, 50% of respondents in France judge friendship to be indispensable. Most of the participants in this survey believe that friendship, like family, allows them to share moments of joy and happiness, as well as more difficult times when they need support.

Friendship is real when it is based on certain values, such as mutual respect, reciprocity, equality, trust and loyalty, in spite of the passage of time and challenging situations. In general, people tend to have few true friends: they can be counted on one hand. Having said that, it is obviously possible to become friendly with a greater number of people, who you may see less regularly but who also help to give your life a sense of balance.

HAVE CONFIDENCE IN YOURSELF

The best way to connect with other people is to learn to have confidence in yourself. Everyone is capable of making friends if they want to, as humans are social by nature.

Many of the people you come across every day struggle with relationships too, even if they try to hide it. Start by being aware that you are not alone in this situation; this will stop you from feeling isolated and worthless. If you need proof of this, all you have to do is look at the number of websites that exist for meeting friends and the community that sustains them. These sites can of course initially help you to prove to yourself that you can get out and meet people, without too much commitment. They will allow you to get in touch with people who live near you and who share the same interests. These platforms are generally free and well designed. When you feel more comfortable with a person, all you have to do is suggest going out (for example to an exhibition, a restaurant, a show or a party).

Talk to other people

To gradually regain confidence in yourself and encourage conversation, start by talking to other people about uncontroversial everyday subjects. Do this at every chance you get, without trying to take the conversation any further.

For example, the next time you are in a shop, put your fear of being rejected to one side and strike up a conversation about the weather. Generally, the staff will be happy to talk to you, especially if you are friendly. You should also make the effort to introduce yourself to your neighbours; more often than not, you will be warmly welcomed. Of course, to do this you will need to be a little braver and bolder to overcome your shyness, but, once again, the results will be worth it.

If you have children, starting a conversation with other parents when you are waiting to pick your child up from school or during extracurricular activities is a good approach. In addition, you could try going to school meetings for parents.

When talking to other people seems more natural to you, be a little more daring. When you run into your neighbour, you could, for example, ask about their children (what are their names? How old are they?). You could also do things like watching a match at a sports bar or seeing an improv show. Try to go regularly to the same public place, as this will give you the chance to run into the same people. If the conditions are right, you will have interesting conversations with nice people, and you will gradually become friendly with them.

You may prefer to avoid people that you do not know at all because this makes you too uncomfortable. If this applies to you, you can start by focusing on people you already know a bit and get along with (colleagues, acquaintances, friends of friends, and so on). Sometimes, all you need to do to make friends is take a step towards the people around you. You do, however, need to take your courage in both hands the first few times to suggest exchanging phone numbers or email addresses.

Make yourself likeable

In all circumstances, try to keep smiling and be casual and cheerful when you talk. This will transmit a positive image of you and encourage the other person to connect with you. According to the American writer Dale Carnegie, author of the bestselling book *How to Win Friends and Influence People*, "a smile says 'I like you. You make me happy. I am glad to see you'" (2006: 69). Try to maintain this cheerfulness as much as possible when you are talking to other people, whether in person or over the phone.

WORK ON YOUR SMILE

As smiling is a vital part of human interaction, do not hesitate to look at how you smile in a mirror. Your smile should be broad, sincere and spontaneous. Avoid rigid smiles, which risk having the opposite effect to the one you were counting on. Be genuine!

You should also make sure to look the person you are speaking to in the eye. Above all, remember the importance of eye contact and do not try to avoid it.

The way you hold yourself is also crucial, as it contributes to the image you convey of yourself. If you slouch, with your shoulders hunched over, this is a more or less clear indication that you lack self-confidence. Correct your posture and try to stand up straight, without seeming awkward.

Once you have followed these first pieces of advice to strike up conversations with people and overcome your initial interpersonal difficulties, you are ready to move on to the following methods.

MAKE CONNECTIONS

Reach out to other people

It is easier to start by approaching just one person, rather than trying to join an established group. Depending on the context, you could ask the person how they are doing or talk about a passion you share. For example, if you are coming out of a meeting, you could mention some of the points brought up in the meeting.

For a healthy conversation to take place, you must be prepared to listen to the other person. You need to listen attentively and encourage the person to talk about themselves, their family or their hobbies. Take a real interest in what they are saying and show that you are interested. To do this, put yourself in their shoes and try to feel what they are feeling. This is known as active listening. When you ask someone how they are doing, be sincere and take a genuine interest in their answer. Avoid simply asking this question as a reflex.

Make the conversation flow more easily by asking open questions, and use the other person's answers to ask more questions. Be empathetic and do not judge; try to accept the other person as they are. Make sure that you do not interrupt them to outdo their story with one of your own. Wait for them to finish what they are saying before you respond and express the idea that you wanted to put forward.

Avoid going off on a tangent. If the person is talking to you about serious things or things that they care a lot about and you immediately change the subject, this will generally give the impression that you are not listening carefully, or even that you are not interested in them.

spontaneity out of your conversation. However, the suggestions below could make it easier to talk to other people.

You could talk about classic, everyday topics such as:

- The weather. The English are particularly fond of talking about the weather, and this can quickly lead to more personal topics, such as weather-dependent activities or outings.
- Holidays. This will allow you to talk about your memories, good places to visit, activities that you particularly enjoyed, and so on.
- Children (especially if you are a parent yourself).
- The news. You should, however, be careful with some potentially riskier topics, such as politics, religion and money.

Find people who share your interests

To make conversation easier, the ideal is to find people who are around the same age as you and who share your interests. The formula to find these lucky few is fairly simple: you need to take part in activities that you enjoy and that are likely to bring together people who share the same passion.

Sport is a good way of doing this. Ideally, this will be a team sport, but other sports can work too. Some individual sports will give you the chance to meet "opponents" (in particular racquet sports, where you can also play doubles matches). Martial arts can also be an interesting way of sharing a particular mindset.

If sport is not for you, do not lose heart. There are many other activities out there, including interests as varied as singing in a choir, pottery, wine tasking courses, cooking classes and photography classes. Any cultural activity that interests you and that you can do in your area is a good option.

You can also get involved with charities or other organisations. Volunteering is another good way of meeting people who share your values and who you will undoubtedly have plenty to talk about with.

Get to know people

When you meet someone, it is very important to memorise their name, because this shows that you are interested in them and remember them, and because it will spare you the embarrassment of having to ask them to refresh your memory. Make it a reflex to introduce yourself at the start of the conversation, which will generally lead the other person to do the same.

If you join a sports team or an association, you will soon

have the chance to exchange phone numbers and email addresses. If the opportunity does not present itself, give out your details to encourage the people you get on well with to do the same. This information can prove very useful if your relationship develops. Let them know that they should feel free to contact you if they want.

If you know the person's birthday, set a reminder on your phone and do not forget to wish them happy birthday. If you do not know it or have simply forgotten, Carnegie suggests a technique to find it out: ask the person if they believe that star signs have an impact on our personality. Very often, the person will end up telling you their sign and their birthday!

To get to know someone better, you need to find out what they like. Try to learn about their other interests (besides the ones that you have in common and that allowed you to meet). You can do this by asking them questions to encourage them to talk about themselves and what interests them.

If you struggle to start a conversation, a helpful and risk-free way to get started is to talk to the organisers of the activity you are taking part in. Offer to help out and let them know when you are available. If they want your help, not only will you get to know the organisers, but you will have more motivation – and even a sense of obligation – to attend regularly. People will naturally approach you because you are part of the team, and you will quickly meet plenty of people.

Show your personality

Once you have started a conversation or once you have got to know the other person a bit better, do not hesitate to talk about yourself, while making sure that you do not make yourself the main topic of conversation. You cannot start a genuine relationship based on a monologue. Talk about your family and your personal life, without going into too much detail. This will give the other person a glimpse of your personality and show them that trust is being established between you. This will allow the other person to feel at ease, and enable your relationship to develop.

MAKE PEOPLE LIKE YOU

Respect differences of opinion

To make others like you, it is very important to respect the opinions of people who you do not necessarily agree with. You therefore need to be open-minded and willing to listen to ideas that do not match your own, without shutting yourself up in your own convictions and beliefs. If you disagree, try to understand the other person's point of view and have a calm discussion without creating tension around the subject. Listen to the other person's arguments and, if you realise that you are wrong, acknowledge it straight away. If you are receptive to new ideas, you can meet people who could change your life.

Highlight your good points and your minor flaws

If you want to come across as likeable, you will of course need to highlight your qualities, meaning the characteristics that give a positive image of you. For example, if you have a good sense of humour, make the most of it: this is an excellent asset. However, make sure you avoid humorous anecdotes about particular groups, as these may not go over well! Similarly, if you know a lot about a particular subject, subtly show it; this might lead people to ask you questions about it. The important thing is to unobtrusively showcase your best features, without coming across as conceited.

You can also mention some of your minor flaws, such as your weakness for food, your tendency to daydream or your clumsiness (without overdoing it), as this can make you more likeable to people. Being sincere will allow them to feel comfortable with you.

In any case, be yourself in every situation. If you are trying to make real friends, people need to like you for who you are and not for the image you are trying to put across. In this case, they may feel tricked when they discover the real you.

Spend time together

For a relationship to develop out of the first conversations, you need to have time to devote to other people. This is generally quite easy if you met at a sports club or an organisation that holds regular meetings. Nonetheless, you should try and plan to see each other outside this setting a few times.

If you feel up to it, invite the person out for a drink, or suggest doing something one evening or weekend (such as hiking, going to the cinema or going jogging). This is assuming that you know a bit about what the person enjoys and that you share the same interests. For example, if you are a member of a football club and support the same team, why not arrange to go watch a match together? If the other person makes the first move, remember to invite them somewhere in return later on.

When you get on well with someone and enjoy talking to them, spending time together and discussing a range of subjects, including personal matters, you can expect this relationship to turn into a real friendship. This can develop gradually over time, as people get to know and like one another, or it can happen very quickly if the two people have a lot in common and click straight away.

SOME ATTITUDES TO ADOPT TO DEVELOP FRIENDSHIPS

- Try to stay positive. People generally feel more comfortable with people who look on the bright side. Similarly, avoid contradicting or criticising other people with negative comments. These are always unpleasant for the other person and make you come across badly.
- Avoid making people repeat things that they have already told you and that you should have remembered.
- Make sure you remember occasions that are im-

portant to the other person.
- If you make jokes, make sure it is clear that you are joking. Not everyone has the same sense of humour, and some jokes could be taken the wrong way or upset someone, even if that was not your intention.
- Do not judge people without getting to know them first. Wait until you have found out a bit more about them before you form an opinion (and even in this case, be prepared for your opinion to change; remember that everyone is developing constantly, you included).
- Encourage people and be there for them during both the good times and the bad.
- Avoid showing up late when you have arranged to meet. While some people will not take exception to you being a few minutes late, others will be frustrated, so you should do everything in your power to be on time. If you are going to be late, always let the other person know and apologise.
- In general, when you say that you are going to do something, make sure that you actually do it. This is the best way to get people to trust you and show that you are reliable.

You will have made a true friend if you both know that you can count on the other person in your hour of need. The real friends are the ones who will still be there during the bad times. You must be prepared to give your time and energy if the other person needs it.

HOW CAN YOU KEEP YOUR FRIENDS?

For a friendship to stand the test of time, you need to work on it. As each person has their own personality and outlook on relationships, some of your friends will need to see you very regularly to maintain this bond, while others will not mind if you only see each other a few times per year. It is up to you to adapt to devote time to each of your friends according to their needs and their idea of friendship.

GOOD HABITS TO ADOPT

Try not to always let the other person call first. Pick up the phone or send a text to catch up or say hi from time to time. The idea is to keep up with what your friends are doing and remind them that you are there.

Friendship should be a two-way street, so if someone does something for you, do not hesitate to return the favour. If you are invited to a dinner with friends, make plans to invite friends over as well. It is much better to go see each other rather than always waiting for someone else to invite you. Similarly, take the initiative to plan quality time with friends: you could go to the cinema, eat out, do a sport, go to an adventure park, go paintballing or simply go out for a drink.

Wish people happy birthday and do not hesitate to get them a small gift; this is one of the things that distinguishes true friends from acquaintances. You could even organise a surprise party. You should also be there on special occasions (weddings, births, baptisms, and so on). Try to mark the occasion and demonstrate your friendship.

You also need to make yourself available when things are going badly, for example during a bereavement, a break-up or an illness. If your friends need you, show them that you are up to the task and that they are a priority for you.

Additionally, if you have a true friend, they may confide in you. Obviously, you need to keep what they have told you to yourself and never tell anyone else. Your friends have to know that they can trust you. In return, you should be able to trust your friends completely and confide in them about the things that are important to you.

Humans are fundamentally social animals, so friendship is essential for their personal fulfilment. For some people, it is one of life's greatest gifts, because it is based on values such as respect and trust. It makes us feel safe and increases our self-confidence, and allows us to feel loved and be ourselves in relationships with other people. Feeling as though we have loyal friends around us contributes to our happiness and gives us a different outlook on life.

FAQS

IS IT EASY TO MAKE FRIENDS?

Making friends is not too difficult once you know how to maximise your chances of developing your relationships. After you meet people and take a liking to them, you need to get closer to them by listening carefully to them and making sure that you come across as likeable and open. You will quickly see which people you can become friends with and, in doing so, realise that making friends is relatively easy.

IS SHYNESS AN OBSTACLE TO FRIENDSHIP?

Shyness can be an obstacle to friendship insofar as it prevents the shy person from approaching people and being open to them. Apart from some people who will naturally make a move towards these shy or isolated individuals, most of the time it will be up to the shy people to reach out to others. Shyness can also be a problem if the person remains withdrawn during a conversation. It is nonetheless important to keep in mind that shyness is not a flaw to overcome, but simply a way of being that needs to be kept in check to stop it from becoming an obstacle.

As such, if you want to make friends, it is essential to learn how to control your shyness. Overcoming this fear of judgement will only make you happier. At the same time, make sure that you still know how to listen, as listening is one of the keys to friendship.

WHAT ARE THE MAIN OBSTACLES STOPPING US FROM MAKING FRIENDS?

Apart from shyness, some elements make it more difficult to make new friends. These include criticising people behind their backs, as this could make people reluctant to trust you. Likewise, making inappropriate jokes will make the people you are talking to feel uncomfortable around you. However, most of the time the thing that really holds us back is not listening to what others have to say and always bringing the conversation back to ourselves, as though things involving us are always better or more important than what the other person is saying to us.

WHAT ARE SOME TIPS TO MAKE NEW FRIENDS?

To make people like you, the first thing you need to do is be friendly. As a general rule, smiling makes you more approachable. Listen and pay attention to what other people say to you. From time to time, talk a bit about yourself so that they can get to know you better and you can develop a deeper relationship. Do not hesitate to compliment people, as long as you really mean what you say. Finally, spending time with people and regularly taking part in activities together will allow you to become closer to them and make real friends.

WHERE CAN I MEET NEW FRIENDS?

Sporting, cultural and voluntary activities will undoubtedly give you the most opportunities to make friends. If you take part in a sport, especially a team sport, you will not be able to avoid sharing experiences with the other person and will have to count on them. On the other hand, cultural or voluntary activities will allow you to meet people who share your interests or values.

IS IT POSSIBLE TO MAKE AND KEEP FRIENDS IF I MOVE A LOT?

When you move house, it is normal to take some time to establish relationships in your new environment. Once you have found your feet, do what you need to do to maximise your chances of making friends and get out and meet people.

If you move a lot but want to maintain the friendships you have developed, you will need to reach out to your friends often, go visit them from time to time, and invite them to come to see you for a few days every now and again. For example, you could meet up by organising holidays together or by getting together on big days like New Year's Eve.

HOW CAN I KEEP MY NEW FRIENDS?

It is vital to maintain your friendships through small acts of kindness. Little things like sending a postcard when you are on holiday and catching up from time to time are important, otherwise you risk not being there when your friends need you. Finally, your real friends should regularly be kept up to date with any big developments or changes in your life.

We want to hear from you!
Leave a comment on your online library
and share your favourite books on social media!

FURTHER READING

BIBLIOGRAPHY

- Carnegie, D. (2006) *How to Win Friends and Influence People*. London: Vermilion.
- Kant, E. (1996) Metaphysical first principles of the doctrine of virtue. In: *The Metaphysics of Morals*. Cambridge: Cambridge University Press.
- Plateau, F. (2015) *Journée mondiale de l'amitié : c'est quoi l'amitié en 2015 ?* [Online]. [Accessed 1 June 2016]. Available from: <http://www.magazine-avantages.fr/,journee-mondiale-de-l-amitie-c-est-quoi-l-amitie-en-2015,183841.asp>

ADDITIONAL SOURCES

- Fine, D. (2006) *The Fine Art Of Small Talk: How to start a conversation in any situation*. London: Piaktus.
- Lowndes, L. (2014) *How to Talk to Anyone: 92 Little Tricks for Big Success in Relationships*. London: Element.
- De Montaigne, M. (2004) *On Friendship*. London: Penguin.

www.50minutes.com

Ebook EAN: 9782806299895

Paperback EAN: 9782806299901

Legal Deposit: D/2017/12603/405

Cover: © Primento

Digital conception by Primento, the digital partner of publishers.

Made in the USA
Monee, IL
07 July 2026